Mind diet

Table of Contents

Introduction

The mind diet is designed to reduce the risk of dementia and loss of brain function as you age.

The mind diet combines the mediterranean diet and the dash diet to create a dietary pattern that focuses specifically on brain health.

What is the mind diet?

"mind" stands for "mediterranean-dash intervention for neurodegenerative delay."

The mind diet aims to reduce dementia and the decline in brain health that often occurs as people get older. It combines aspects of two very popular diets, the mediterranean diet and the dietary approaches to stop hypertension (dash) diet.

Many experts regard the mediterranean and dash diets as two of the healthiest diets.

Research has shown that they can lower blood pressure and reduce the risk of heart disease, diabetes, and several other diseases. But researchers wanted to create a diet specifically to help improve brain function and prevent dementia.

To do this, they combined foods from the mediterranean and dash diets that had been shown to benefit brain health. For example, the mediterranean and dash diets both recommend eating a lot of fruit. Fruit intake has been linked with improved brain function, but berries in particular are supported by the strongest evidence.

Thus, the mind diet encourages eating berries but does not emphasize consuming fruit in general.

Currently, there are no set guidelines for how to follow the mind diet. You can simply eat more of the 10 foods that the diet encourages and eat less of the 5 foods that it recommends you limit.

10 foods to eat on the mind diet

Here are the 10 foods the mind diet encourages:

- **Green, leafy vegetables:** aim for six or more servings per week. This includes kale, spinach, cooked greens, and salads.
- **All other vegetables:** try to eat another vegetable in addition to the green leafy vegetables at least once per day. It's best to choose non-starchy vegetables because they provide a lot of nutrients for a low number of calories.
- **Berries:** eat berries at least twice per week. Berries such as strawberries, blueberries, raspberries, and blackberries all have antioxidant benefits.

- **Nuts**: try to get five or more servings of nuts each week. The creators of the mind diet don't specify what kind of nuts to consume, but it is probably best to vary the type of nuts you eat to obtain a variety of nutrients.

- **Olive oil:** use olive oil as your main cooking oil. Check out this article for information about the safety of cooking with olive oil.

- **Whole grains**: aim for at least three servings daily. Choose whole grains like oatmeal, quinoa, brown rice, whole wheat pasta, and 100% whole wheat bread.

- **Fish**: eat fish at least once per week. It is best to choose fatty fish such as salmon, sardines, trout, tuna, and mackerel for their high amounts of omega-3 fatty acids.

- **Beans**: include beans in at least four meals per week. This category includes all beans, lentils, and soybeans.

- **Poultry**: try to eat chicken or turkey at least twice per week. Note that fried chicken is not encouraged on the mind diet.

- **Wine**: aim for no more than one glass daily. Both red and white wine may benefit your brain. While there has been much interest in the compound resveratrol, which is found in red wine, recent research has questioned whether it has clear benefits in humans.

If you're unable to consume the target number of servings, don't quit the mind diet altogether. Research has shown that following the mind diet even to a moderate degree is associated with a reduced risk of alzheimer's disease and cognitive impairment.

5 foods to avoid on the mind diet

The mind diet recommends limiting the following five foods:

- **Butter and margarine:** try to eat less than 1 tablespoon (about 14 grams) daily. Instead, try using olive oil as your primary cooking fat and dipping your bread in olive oil with herbs.

- **Cheese**: the mind diet recommends eating cheese less than once per week.

- **Red meat**: aim for no more than three servings per week. This category includes all beef, pork, lamb, and products made from these meats.

- **Fried food**: the mind diet highly discourages fried food, especially the kind from fast-food restaurants. Limit your consumption to less than once per week.

- **Pastries and sweets**: this includes most of the processed snack foods and desserts you may think of — ice cream, cookies, brownies, snack cakes, doughnuts, candy, and more. Try to limit these to no more than four times per week.

Researchers encourage limiting your consumption of these foods because they contain saturated fats.

Studies have found that trans fats are clearly associated with all sorts of diseases, including heart disease and even alzheimer's disease. However, the health effects of saturated fat are widely debated in the nutrition world.

It's worth noting that partially hydrogenated oils (the major source of trans fats in the food supply) have been banned by the fda since 2020. They're still naturally found in much lower amounts in fried foods, dairy, or red meat, but margarine, pastries, and sweets are no longer a major source.

Although the research on saturated fats and heart disease may be inconclusive and highly contested, animal research and observational studies in humans do suggest that consuming saturated fats in excess is associated with poor brain health.

The mind diet may decrease oxidative stress and inflammation

The current research on the mind diet has not been able to determine exactly how the diet works. However, scientists think it may work by reducing oxidative stress and inflammation .

Oxidative stress occurs when unstable molecules called free radicals accumulate in the body in large amounts. This often causes damage to cells. The brain is especially vulnerable to this type of damage.

Inflammation is your body's natural response to injury and infection. But if it's not properly regulated, inflammation can also be harmful and contribute to many chronic diseases.

Together, oxidative stress and inflammation can be quite detrimental to your brain. In recent years, they have been the focus of some interventions to prevent and treat alzheimer's disease.

Following the mediterranean and dash diets has been associated with lower levels of oxidative stress and inflammation.

Because the mind diet is a hybrid of these two diets, the foods that make up the mind diet probably also have antioxidant and anti-inflammatory effects.

The antioxidants in berries and the vitamin e in olive oil, green leafy vegetables, and nuts are thought to benefit brain function by protecting the brain from oxidative stress.

Additionally, the omega-3 fatty acids found in fatty fish are well known for their ability to lower inflammation in the brain and have been associated with slower loss of brain function.

The mind diet may reduce harmful beta-amyloid proteins

Researchers also believe the mind diet may benefit the brain by reducing potentially harmful beta-amyloid proteins. Beta-amyloid proteins are protein fragments found naturally in the body.

However, they can accumulate and form plaques that build up in the brain, disrupting communication between brain cells and eventually leading to brain cell death.

In fact, many scientists believe these plaques are one of the primary causes of alzheimer's disease.

Animal and test-tube studies suggest that the antioxidants that many mind diet foods contain may help prevent the formation of beta-amyloid plaques in the brain.

 additionally, the mind diet limits foods that contain saturated fats and trans fats, which studies have shown can increase beta-amyloid protein levels in the brains of mice. Human observational studies have found that consuming these fats is associated with a doubled risk of alzheimer's disease.

However, it is important to note that this type of research is not able to determine cause and effect. Higher quality, controlled studies are needed to discover exactly how the mind diet may benefit brain health.

Research on the mind diet and brain health

The first official paper on the mind diet was published in 2015. Since then, researchers have performed additional studies to investigate the benefits of the diet for brain health.

Previous observational studies showed that the mind diet was associated with a decreased risk of developing alzheimer's disease as well as slowed cognitive decline

However, both of these studies were observational, which means they cannot indicate cause and effect — they can only detect associations.

More recently, a 2021 study found that the mind diet slowed the rate of cognitive decline in people who had experienced a stroke.

Additionally, a 2022 study found that middle-aged adults who closely adhered to the mind diet had faster information processing speeds than those who did not closely follow the diet.

A 2022 randomized clinical trial in 50 healthy obese women found that those who followed a calorie-restricted mind diet for 3 months had higher scores for working memory, verbal recognition memory, and attention compared to the calorie-restricted control group. That said, more research is still needed to gauge the true effectiveness of the mind diet. A new clinical trial is in progress.

Best foods to boost your brain and memory

Foods that are good for your brain can help keep this crucial organ healthy and can improve your ability to do specific mental tasks, such as memory and concentration.

Your brain is kind of a big deal. As the control center of your body, it's in charge of keeping your heart beating and lungs breathing and allowing you to move, feel, and think. That's why eating certain foods can help you keep your brain in peak working condition.

Fatty fish

When people talk about brain foods, fatty fish is often at the top of the list. This type of fish includes salmon, trout, albacore tuna, herring, and sardines, all of which are rich sources of omega-3 fatty acids. About 60% of your brain is made of fat, and half of that fat is comprised of omega-3 fatty acids.

Your brain uses omega-3s to build brain and nerve cells, and these fats are essential for learning and memory. Omega-3s also offer several additional benefits for your brain.

For one thing, they may slow age-related mental decline and help ward off alzheimer's disease. On the flip side, not getting enough omega-3s is linked to learning impairments, as well as depression. In general, eating fish seems to have positive health benefits.

Coffee

If coffee is the highlight of your morning, you'll be glad to hear that it's good for you. Two main components in coffee — caffeine and antioxidants — can help support brain health.

the caffeine found in coffee has a number of positive effects on the brain, including:

- **Increased alertness**. Caffeine keeps your brain alert by blocking adenosine, a chemical messenger that makes you feel sleepy.

- **Improved mood**. Caffeine may also boost some of your "feel-good" neurotransmitters, such as dopamine.

- **Sharpened concentration**. One study found that caffeine consumption led to short-term improvements in attention and alertness in participants completing a cognition test.

Drinking coffee over the long-term is also linked to a reduced risk of neurological diseases, such as parkinson's and alzheimer's. The largest risk reduction was seen in those adults who consumes 3-4 cups daily. This could at least be partly due to coffee's high concentration of antioxidants.

Blueberries

Blueberries provide numerous health benefits, including some that are specifically for your brain. Blueberries and other deeply colored berries deliver anthocyanins, a group of plant compounds with anti-inflammatory and antioxidant effects.

Antioxidants act against both oxidative stress and inflammation, conditions that can contribute to brain aging and neurodegenerative diseases. Some of the antioxidants in blueberries have been found to accumulate in the brain and help improve communication between brain cells.

According to one review of 11 studies, blueberries could help improve memory and certain cognitive processes in children and older adults.

Turmeric

Turmeric has generated a lot of buzz recently. This deep-yellow spice is a key ingredient in curry powder and has a number of benefits for the brain.

Curcumin, the active ingredient in turmeric, has been shown to cross the blood-brain barrier, meaning it can directly enter the brain and benefit the cells there. It's a potent antioxidant and anti-inflammatory compound that has been linked to the following brain benefits:

- **May benefit memory**. Curcumin may help improve memory in people with alzheimer's. It may also help clear the

amyloid plaques that are a hallmark of
this disease.

- **Eases depression**. Curcumin boosts
serotonin and dopamine, both of which
improve mood. One review found that
curcumin could improve symptoms of
depression and anxiety when used
alongside standard treatments in people
diagnosed with depression.

- **Helps new brain cells grow**. Curcumin
boosts brain-derived neurotrophic factor,
a type of growth hormone that helps
brain cells grow. It may help delay age-
related mental decline, but more research
is needed.

Therefore, while adding turmeric to your food
may be beneficial, you may need to use a
curcumin supplement under a doctor's guidance
to obtain the results reported in these studies.

Broccoli

Broccoli is packed with powerful plant compounds, including antioxidants. It's also very high in vitamin k, delivering more than 100% of the recommended daily intake (rdi) in a 1-cup (160-gram) serving of cooked broccoli.

This fat-soluble vitamin is essential for forming sphingolipids, a type of fat that's densely packed into brain cells.

Beyond vitamin k, broccoli contains a number of compounds that give it anti-inflammatory and antioxidant effects, which may help protect the brain against damage.

Pumpkin seeds

Pumpkin seeds contain powerful antioxidants that protect the body and brain from free-radical damage. They're also an excellent source of magnesium, iron, zinc, and copper. Each of these nutrients is important for brain health:

- **Zinc**. This element is crucial for nerve signaling. Zinc deficiency has been linked to many neurological conditions, including alzheimer's disease, depression, and parkinson's disease

- **Magnesium**. Magnesium is essential for learning and memory. Low magnesium levels are linked to many neurological diseases, including migraine, depression, and epilepsy

- **Copper**. Your brain uses copper to help control nerve signals. And when copper levels are out of whack, there's a higher risk of neurodegenerative disorders, such as alzheimer's.

- **Iron**. Iron deficiency is often characterized by brain fog and impaired brain function

The research focuses mostly on these micronutrients, rather than pumpkin seeds themselves. However, since pumpkin seeds are high in these micronutrients, you can likely reap their benefits by adding pumpkin seeds to your diet.

Dark chocolate

Dark chocolate and cocoa powder are packed with a few brain-boosting compounds, including flavonoids, caffeine, and antioxidants.

Dark chocolate has a 70% or greater cocoa content. These benefits are not seen with regular milk chocolate, which contains between 10–50% cocoa. Flavonoids are a group of antioxidant plant compounds.

the flavonoids in chocolate gather in the areas of the brain that deal with learning and memory. Researchers believe that these compounds may enhance memory and also help slow down age-related mental decline.

Nuts

Research has shown that eating nuts can improve heart-health markers, and having a healthy heart is linked to having a healthy brain.

One study found that regular consumption of nuts could be linked to a lower risk of cognitive decline in older adults. Also, another 2014 study found that women who ate nuts regularly over the course of several years had a sharper memory compared with those who did not eat nuts.

Several nutrients in nuts, such as healthy fats, antioxidants, and vitamin e, may explain their beneficial effects on brain health. Vitamin e protects cells against free-radical damage to help slow mental decline.

While all nuts are good for your brain, walnuts may have an extra edge, since they also deliver anti-inflammatory omega-3 fatty acids.

Oranges

You can get almost all the vitamin c you need in a day by eating one medium orange. Doing so is important for brain health since vitamin c is a key factor in preventing mental decline.

According to one study, having higher levels of vitamin c in the blood was associated with improvements in tasks involving focus, memory, attention, and decision speed.

Vitamin c is a powerful antioxidant that helps fight off the free radicals that can damage brain cells. Plus, vitamin c supports brain health as you age and may protect against conditions like major depressive disorder, anxiety, schizophrenia, and alzheimer's disease. You can also get high amounts of vitamin c from other foods like bell peppers, guava, kiwi, tomatoes, and strawberries.

Eggs

Eggs are a good source of several nutrients tied to brain health, including vitamins b6 and b12, folate, and choline. Choline is an important micronutrient that your body uses to create acetylcholine, a neurotransmitter that helps regulate mood and memory.

 two older studies found that higher intakes of choline were linked to better memory and mental function. Nevertheless, many people do not get enough choline in their diet.

Eating eggs is an easy way to get choline, given that egg yolks are among the most concentrated sources of this nutrient. Adequate intake of choline is 425 mg per day for most women and 550 mg per day for men, with just a single egg yolk containing 112 mg.

Furthermore, the b vitamins found in eggs also have several roles in brain health.

To start, they may help slow the progression of mental decline in older adults by lowering levels of homocysteine, an amino acid that could be linked to dementia and alzheimer's disease.

The 7 worst foods for your brain

Consuming unhealthy foods, alcohol, and fish with mercury can negatively affect cognitive function. While you don't have to avoid these things completely, it's a good idea to limit them. Opt for a diet with whole, fresh foods to better support brain health.

Your brain is the most important organ in your body. It keeps your heart beating, lungs breathing and all the systems in your body functioning.

that's why it's essential to keep your brain working in optimum condition with a healthy diet. Some foods have negative effects on the brain, impacting your memory and mood and increasing your risk of dementia. Estimates predict that dementia will affect more than 65 million people worldwide by 2030.

luckily, you can help reduce your risk of the disease by cutting certain foods out of your diet.

Sugary drinks

Sugary drinks include beverages like soda, sports drinks, energy drinks and fruit juice. A high intake of sugary drinks not only expands your waistline and boosts your risk of type 2 diabetes and heart disease — it also has a negative effect on your brain

In addition, higher sugar levels in the blood can increase the risk of dementia, even in people without diabetes. A primary component of many sugary drinks is high-fructose corn syrup (hfcs), which consists of 55% fructose and 45% glucose. A high intake of fructose can lead to obesity, high blood pressure, high blood fats, diabetes and arterial dysfunction. These aspects of metabolic syndrome may lead to an increase in the long-term risk of developing dementia.

Animal studies have shown that a high fructose intake can lead to insulin resistance in the brain, as well as a reduction in brain function, memory, learning and the formation of brain neurons.

While further studies in humans are needed, the results suggest that a high intake of fructose from sugary drinks may have additional negative effects on the brain, beyond the effects of sugar.

Some alternatives to sugary drinks include water, unsweetened iced tea, vegetable juice and unsweetened dairy products.

refined carbs

Refined carbohydrates include sugars and highly processed grains, such as white flour.

These types of carbs generally have a high glycemic index (gi). This means your body digests them quickly, causing a spike in your blood sugar and insulin levels.

Also, when eaten in larger quantities, these foods often have a high glycemic load (gl). The gl refers to how much a food raises your blood sugar levels, based on the serving size.

Foods that are high-gi and high-gl have been found to impair brain function. Research has shown that just a single meal with a high glycemic load can impair memory in both children and adults.

Another study in healthy university students found that those who had a higher intake of fat and refined sugar also had poorer memory.

This effect on memory may be due to inflammation of the hippocampus, a part of the brain that affects some aspects of memory, as well as responsiveness to hunger and fullness cues. Inflammation is recognized as a risk factor for degenerative diseases of the brain, including alzheimer's disease and dementia.

Foods high in trans fats

Trans fats are a type of unsaturated fat that can have a detrimental effect on brain health. While trans fats occur naturally in animal products like meat and dairy, these are not a major concern. It's industrially produced trans fats, also known as hydrogenated vegetable oils, that are a problem.

These artificial trans fats can be found in shortening, margarine, frosting, snack foods, ready-made cakes and prepackaged cookies.

Studies have found that when people consume higher amounts of trans fats, they tend to have an increased risk of alzheimer's disease, poorer memory, lower brain volume and cognitive decline.

However, some studies have not found an association between trans-fat intake and brain health. Nonetheless, trans fats should be avoided. They have a negative effect on many other aspects of health, including heart health and inflammation.

The evidence on saturated fat is mixed. Three observational studies have found a positive association between saturated fat intake and the risk of alzheimer's disease, whereas a fourth study showed the opposite effect.

One cause for this may be that a subset of the test populations had a genetic susceptibility to the disease, which is caused by a gene known as apoe4. However, more research is required on this topic.

Highly processed foods

Highly processed foods tend to be high in sugar, added fats and salt. They include foods such as chips, sweets, instant noodles, microwave popcorn, store-bought sauces and ready-made meals.

These foods are usually high in calories and low in other nutrients. They're exactly the kinds of foods that cause weight gain, which can have a negative effect on your brain health.

A study in 243 people found increased fat around the organs, or visceral fat, is associated with brain tissue damage. Another study in 130 people found there's a measurable decrease in brain tissue even in the early stages of metabolic syndrome.

The nutrient composition of processed foods in the western diet can also negatively affect the brain and contribute to the development of degenerative diseases. A study including 52 people found that a diet high in unhealthy ingredients resulted in lower levels of sugar metabolism in the brain and a decrease in brain tissue. These factors are thought to be markers for alzheimer's disease.

Highly processed foods

Highly processed foods tend to be high in sugar, added fats and salt. They include foods such as chips, sweets, instant noodles, microwave popcorn, store-bought sauces and ready-made meals.

These foods are usually high in calories and low in other nutrients. They're exactly the kinds of foods that cause weight gain, which can have a negative effect on your brain health.

A study in 243 people found increased fat around the organs, or visceral fat, is associated with brain tissue damage. Another study in 130 people found there's a measurable decrease in brain tissue even in the early stages of metabolic syndrome.

The nutrient composition of processed foods in the western diet can also negatively affect the brain and contribute to the development of degenerative diseases.

One of the ways processed foods may negatively impact the brain is by reducing the production of a molecule called brain-derived neurotrophic factor (bdnf). This molecule is found in various parts of the brain, including the hippocampus, and it's important for long-term memory, learning and the growth of new neurons. Therefore, any reduction can have negative impacts on these functions.

You can avoid processed foods by eating mostly fresh, whole foods such as fruits, vegetables, nuts, seeds, legumes, meat and fish. Additionally, a mediterranean-style diet has been shown to protect against cognitive decline.

Aspartame

Aspartame is an artificial sweetener used in many sugar-free products. People often choose to use it when trying to lose weight or avoid sugar when they have diabetes. It is also found in many commercial products not specifically targeted at people with diabetes.

However, this widely used sweetener has also been linked to behavioral and cognitive problems, though the research has been controversial. Aspartame is made of phenylalanine, methanol and aspartic acid.

Phenylalanine can cross the blood-brain barrier and might disrupt the production of neurotransmitters. Additionally, aspartame is a chemical stressor and may increase the brain's vulnerability to oxidative stress.

Alcohol

When consumed in moderation, alcohol can be an enjoyable addition to a nice meal. However, excessive consumption can have serious effects on the brain.

Chronic alcohol use results in a reduction in brain volume, metabolic changes and disruption of neurotransmitters, which are chemicals the brain uses to communicate. People with alcoholism often have a deficiency in vitamin b1. This can lead to a brain disorder called wernicke's encephalopathy, which in turn can develop into korsakoff's syndrome.

This syndrome is distinguished by severe damage to the brain, including memory loss, disturbances in eyesight, confusion and unsteadiness. Excessive consumption of alcohol can also have negative effects in non-alcoholics.

Heavy one-off drinking episodes are known as "binge drinking." These acute episodes can cause the brain to interpret emotional cues differently than normal. For example, people have a reduced sensitivity to sad faces and an increased sensitivity to angry faces. It's thought that these changes to emotion recognition may be a cause of alcohol-related aggression.

Fish high in mercury

Mercury is a heavy metal contaminant and neurological poison that can be stored for a long time in animal tissues.

Long-lived, predatory fish are particularly susceptible to accumulating mercury and can carry amounts over 1 million times the concentration of their surrounding water. For this reason, the primary food source of mercury in humans is seafood, particularly wild varieties.

After a person ingests mercury, it spreads all around their body, concentrating in the brain, liver and kidneys. In pregnant women, it also concentrates in the placenta and fetus.

The effects of mercury toxicity include disruption of the central nervous system and neurotransmitters and stimulation of neurotoxins, resulting in damage to the brain.

For developing fetuses and young children, mercury can disrupt brain development and cause the destruction of cell components. This can lead to cerebral palsy and other developmental delays and deficits.

However, most fish are not a significant source of mercury. In fact, fish is a high-quality protein and contains many important nutrients, such as omega-3s, vitamin b12, zinc, iron and magnesium. Therefore, it is important to include fish as part of a healthy diet.

Generally, it is recommended that adults eat two to three servings of fish per week. However, if you're eating shark or swordfish, only consume one serving, and then no other fish that week.

Pregnant women and children should avoid or limit high-mercury fish, including shark, swordfish, tuna, orange roughy, king mackerel and tilefish. However, it's still safe to have two to three servings of other low-mercury fish per week.

Recommendations may differ from country to country, depending on the types of fish in your area, so it's always best to check with your local food safety agency for the recommendations that are right for you. Also, if you are catching your own fish, it is a good idea to check with local authorities about the levels of mercury in the water you are fishing from.

eat less added sugar

Eating too much added sugar has been linked to many health issues and chronic diseases, including cognitive decline.

Research has shown that a sugar-laden diet can lead to poor memory and reduced brain volume, particularly in the area of the brain that stores short-term memory.

For example, one study of more than 4,000 people found that those with a higher intake of sugary beverages like soda had lower total brain volumes and poorer memories on average compared with people who consumed less sugar.

Cutting back on sugar not only helps your memory but also improves your overall health.

try a fish oil supplement

Fish oil is rich in the omega-3 fatty acids eicosapentaenoic acid (epa) and docosahexaenoic acid (dha). These fats are important for overall health and have been shown to lower the risk of heart disease, reduce inflammation, relieve stress and anxiety, and slow mental decline.

Many studies have shown that consuming fish and fish oil supplements may improve memory, especially in older people.

Both dha and epa are vital to the health and functioning of the brain and also help reduce inflammation in the body, which has been linked to cognitive decline.

Make time for meditation

The practice of meditation may positively affect your health in many ways. It is relaxing and soothing, and has been found to reduce stress and pain, lower blood pressure and even improve memory. In fact, meditation has been shown to increase gray matter in the brain. Gray matter contains neuron cell bodies. As you age, gray matter declines, which negatively impacts memory and cognition

Meditation and relaxation techniques have been shown to improve short-term memory in people of all ages, from people in their 20s to older adults. For example, one study showed that taiwanese college students who engaged in meditation practices like mindfulness had significantly better spatial working memory than students who did not practice meditation.

Spatial working memory is the ability to hold and process information in your mind about the positions of objects in space.

Maintain a moderate weight

Maintaining a moderate body weight is essential for well-being and is one of the best ways to keep your body and mind in top condition.

Several studies have established obesity as a risk factor for cognitive decline. Having obesity can actually cause changes to memory-associated genes in the brain, negatively affecting memory.

Obesity can also lead to insulin resistance and inflammation, both of which can negatively impact the brain.

Obesity is also associated with a higher risk of developing alzheimer's disease, a progressive disease that destroys memory and cognitive function.

Practice mindfulness

Mindfulness is a mental state in which you focus on your present situation, maintaining awareness of your surroundings and feelings.

Mindfulness is used in meditation, but the two aren't one and the same. Meditation is a more formal practice, whereas mindfulness is a mental habit you can use in any situation. Studies have shown that mindfulness is effective at lowering stress and improving concentration and memory.

One study of 293 psychology students showed that those who underwent mindfulness training had improved recognition-memory performance when recalling objects compared with students who did not receive mindfulness training.

Mindfulness has also been linked with a lower risk of age-related cognitive decline and an overall improvement in psychological well-being. Incorporate mindfulness techniques into your daily routine by paying more attention to your present situation, concentrating on your breathing, and gently resetting your attention when your mind wanders.

Practice mindfulness

Mindfulness is a mental state in which you focus on your present situation, maintaining awareness of your surroundings and feelings.

Mindfulness is used in meditation, but the two aren't one and the same. Meditation is a more formal practice, whereas mindfulness is a mental habit you can use in any situation.

Studies have shown that mindfulness is effective at lowering stress and improving concentration and memory.

Mindfulness has also been linked with a lower risk of age-related cognitive decline and an overall improvement in psychological well-being.

Incorporate mindfulness techniques into your daily routine by paying more attention to your present situation, concentrating on your breathing, and gently resetting your attention when your mind wanders.

Train your brain

Exercising your cognitive skills by playing brain games is a fun and effective way to boost your memory. Crosswords, word-recall games, tetris, and even mobile apps dedicated to memory training are excellent ways to strengthen memory.

 A study that included 42 adults with mild cognitive impairment found that playing games on a brain-training app for 8 hours over a 4-week period improved performance in memory tests.

Plus, brain-training games have been shown to help reduce the risk of dementia in older adults.

Limit refined carbs

Consuming large amounts of refined carbohydrates like cakes, cereal, cookies, white rice, and white bread may be damaging to your memory.

These foods have a high glycemic index, meaning the body digests these carbohydrates quickly, leading to a spike in blood sugar levels. Studies have shown that the western diet, which is high in refined carbohydrates, is associated with dementia, cognitive decline, and reduced cognitive function.

Another study demonstrated that adults who consumed ready-to-eat breakfast cereal daily had poorer cognitive function than those who consumed cereal less frequently.

Get your vitamin d levels tested

Vitamin d is an important nutrient that plays many vital roles in the body. Low levels of vitamin d have been linked to a host of health issues, including a reduction in cognitive function.

Low levels of vitamin d have also been linked to a greater risk of developing dementia. Vitamin d deficiency is very common, especially in colder climates and in those with darker skin. Speak with your doctor about getting a blood test to find out if you need a vitamin d supplement.

Exercise

Exercise is important for overall physical and mental health. Research has established that it's beneficial for the brain and may help improve memory in people of all ages, from children to older adults.

For example, a study of 144 people aged 19 to 93 showed that a single bout of 15 minutes of moderate exercise on a stationary bike led to improved cognitive performance, including memory, across all ages.

Many studies have shown exercise may increase the secretion of neuroprotective proteins and improve the growth and development of neurons, leading to improved brain health. Regular exercise in midlife is also associated with a decreased risk of developing dementia later in life.

Choose anti-inflammatory foods

Consuming a diet rich in anti-inflammatory foods may help improve your memory.

Antioxidants help lower inflammation in the body by reducing oxidative stress caused by free radicals. You can consume antioxidants in foods like fruits, vegetables, and teas.

A recent review of nine studies with more than 31,000 people found that those who ate more fruits and vegetables had lower risks of cognitive decline and dementia compared to those who consumed less of these nutritious foods

Berries are particularly high in antioxidants like flavonoids and anthocyanins. Eating them may be an excellent way to prevent memory loss.

Consider curcumin

Curcumin is a compound found in high concentrations in turmeric root. It's one of a category of compounds called polyphenols.

It is a potent antioxidant and exerts powerful anti-inflammatory effects in the body.

Studies have found that curcumin reduces oxidative damage and inflammation in the brain and also lowers the quantity of amyloid plaques. These accumulate on neurons and cause cell and tissue death, leading to memory loss.

In fact, amyloid plaque buildup may play a role in the progression of alzheimer's disease.

Though more human studies are needed on the effects of curcumin on memory, some studies suggest it may be effective at boosting memory and preventing cognitive decline.

Add some cocoa to your diet

Cocoa is not only delicious but also nutritious, providing a powerful dose of antioxidants called flavonoids. Research suggests flavonoids are particularly beneficial to the brain.

They may help stimulate the growth of blood vessels and neurons and increase blood flow in parts of the brain involved with memory.

A study of 30 healthy people found that those who consumed dark chocolate containing 720 mg of cocoa flavonoids demonstrated better memory compared to those who consumed white chocolate without cocoa flavonoids

To get the most benefit out of chocolate, choose dark chocolate with a cocoa content of 70% cacao or higher. That will help ensure it contains larger amounts of antioxidants like flavonoids.

Summary

The mind diet was created to help prevent dementia and slow the decline in brain function that can happen with age.

The diet encourages consuming vegetables, berries, nuts, whole grains, olive oil, fish, beans, poultry, and wine.

These foods contain many nutrients that promote good brain health, possibly by reducing oxidative stress, inflammation, and the formation of beta-amyloid plaques.

Because the mind diet is a combination of the mediterranean and dash diets, it will not be surprising if future research shows that it offers other health benefits that are also associated with these two diets.

But for now, if you're looking for a way of eating that focuses on maintaining brain health as you age, the mind diet is a great approach that's simple to follow. There are many fun, simple and even delicious ways to improve your memory.

Exercising your mind and body, enjoying a quality piece of chocolate and reducing the amount of added sugar in your diet are all excellent techniques.

Try adding a few of these science-backed tips to your daily routine to boost your brain health and keep your memory in top condition.

MIND diet recipes

1. **Ground bison breakfast sausage**

Ingredients

- 1 pound ground bison (90/10)

- 2 teaspoons black pepper

- 1 teaspoon kosher salt

- 1 teaspoon smoked paprika

- 1/2 teaspoon crushed red pepper flakes

- 1/2 teaspoon rubbed sage

- 1/4 teaspoon allspice

- 2 tablespoons (30g) maple syrup

Instructions

1. Mix the dry ingredients together in a small bowl and set aside.

2. Pat the ground bison dry with a paper towel and add to a large bowl. Press the bison up the sides of the bowl to maximize surface area. Sprinkle half the seasoning blend over the bison, flip, and season the other side. Gently mix the bison by hand to evenly incorporate the

seasoning blend. Add the maple syrup and gently mix to incorporate.

3. Cover and let the bison rest for 20-30 minutes. (refrigerate overnight for best results.)

4. Divide the bison into 10 portions, weighing about 1.7 ounces (48g) each. Press each portion into thin patties and place on a sheet pan or large plate.

5. To cook, heat a large skillet or griddle over medium heat with 1/2 tablespoon oil or cooking spray. (cooking with too much heat will burn the exterior before the sausage cook through.)

6. Once hot, add the sausage patties and cook for 2-3 minutes until well browned on one side. Flip and cook an additional 2-3 minutes until the sausages reach an internal temperature of 160ºf. (you may

need to cook in batches, depending on the size of your pan.)

2. Toasted coconut mocha frappuccino

Ingredients

- 1 cup strong brewed coffee (chilled // french press or cold brew is best)
- 8 coconut milk ice cubes (or other milk // 3/4 cup full-fat or light coconut milk yields ~8 cubes)*
- 1/4 cup toasted unsweetened coconut flake (plus more for topping)
- 2 tbsp light chocolate syrup (or other chocolate sauce // plus more for topping)
- 1 tbsp cocoa powder

Instructions

1. The night before making, pour your (well-shaken) coconut milk (about 1 can as

original recipe is written) into an ice cube tray. You'll need 8-10 cubes for one drink, and one can yields about one full tray. Save the leftover cubes for another drink.

2. In the morning, toast your coconut by spreading 1/4 on a baking sheet and baking for 3-5 minutes in a 350-degree f (190 c) oven.

3. Next place all ingredients in a blender and mix until smooth and well combined.

4. To thicken, add more coconut ice cubes. To thin, add more coffee or chocolate syrup.

5. Serve immediately, or freeze for later. Top with coconut whipped cream, more toasted coconut and a drizzle of chocolate syrup, if desired. Nutrition does not reflect toppings.

6. Notes

7. *using full-fat coconut milk does add more calories, but it makes the drink much creamier. However, light coconut milk or coconut milk beverage will work fine here, too.

3. **Spinach, goat cheese & chorizo omelette**

Ingredients

- 4 ounces chorizo sausage
- 1/2 tablespoon butter
- 4 eggs
- 1 tablespoon water
- 2 ounces crumbled fresh goat cheese
- 2 cups baby spinach leaves
- Sliced avocado (optional)
- 1/4 cup salsa verde (optional)

Instructions

1. Remove chorizo from the casing and fry in a medium saute pan until fully cooked about 6 – 8 minutes.
2. Meanwhile beat the eggs and water in a small bowl.*
3. Take the chorizo out of the pan with a slotted spoon and set aside. Wipe the pan of the remaining grease with a clean paper towel.
4. Melt the butter in the same pan over low heat.
5. Add the beaten eggs to the pan, then put the chorizo, spinach, and crumbled goat cheese on half the egg mixture.
6. Cook on low heat for 3 minutes until slightly firm, then fold the empty side over the side with the filling on it. Cover the pan with foil or a pot cover and leave on low heat for another 3 minutes until the eggs are cooked through.

7. If your bottom is browning too quickly, turn the stove off and leave the pan covered for up to 10 minutes and the residual heat should "bake" it until the center is fully cooked.

8. Serve with avocado slices and salsa verde. So good you won't even miss the toast or hash browns!

Notes

*as a side note, i add the water because as the egg cooks the water turns to steam which helps the egg puff up and get fluffy. Some people like to add milk or cream and you could do that too – totally a matter of personal preference.

4. Ezekiel french toast

Ingredients

- 2 slices ezekiel bread

- 2 eggs

- 2 tablespoons milk of choice – i used organic skim milk, but almond milk works well too

- 1 tablespoon cinnamon

- 1 teaspoon raw honey (optional)

- 1 teaspoon coconut oil

- Toppings of choice – i used pure maple syrup, and sliced strawberries & bananas

Instructions

1. Heat a non-stick pan over a low to medium. Grease pan with the coconut oil.

2. Scramble the eggs, milk, cinnamon, and honey in a medium bowl. Transfer the egg mixture in a pie dish, or low-set bowl.

3. Dunk the ezekiel bread in the egg mixture for 15 second on each side.

4. Cook the ezekiel bread for 2-3 minutes on each side until golden brown.

5. Serve warm with toppings of choice.

5. Paleo pumpkin and carrot muffins

Ingredients

- 3 large eggs at room temperature
- 4 medium carrots peeled
- 1½ cups finely ground almond flour spooned and leveled
- 1½ teaspoons five spice powder you can substitute pumpkin spice blend
- 1 teaspoons baking soda
- ½ teaspoon cream of tartar
- ½ teaspoon ground cinnamon
- ⅛ teaspoon fine sea salt
- ¾ cup canned pumpkin purée
- ½ cup honey
- 2 tablespoons almond butter

- 1 teaspoon melted coconut oil and a bit extra for greasing the muffin tin if not using paper liners
- 1 tablespoon sliced almonds
- 1 tablespoon toasted pumpkin seeds

Instructions

1. Heat oven to 350°f with the rack in the middle position, and take your eggs out of the fridge. It's important that your eggs are at room temperature when you start blending the liquid ingredients, or things'll get chunky.
2. Line a muffin tin with paper liners.
3. Next, grate your peeled carrots by hand or in a food processor and place the shredded carrots in a doubled piece of cheese cloth or clean dish towel. (trust me: paper towels will tear.) Gather up the sides of the cloth and wring out the excess

carrot juice and set the carrot shreds aside. The final volume of the shredded carrots should be 1½ cups.

4. In a large bowl, whisk together the almond flour, five spice powder, baking soda, cream of tartar, ground cinnamon, and sea salt.

5. In a separate bowl, whisk the eggs well. Mix in the pumpkin, honey, almond butter, and melted coconut oil. (again, make sure these ingredients are at room temperature, or the coconut oil will harden and clump up).

6. Add the wet ingredients to the dry, and stir until combined. Fold in the grated carrots.

7. Scoop the batter evenly into the muffin tins, filling them about ¾ full. Sprinkle sliced almonds and toasted pumpkin

seeds on top before placing the muffins in the oven.

8. Bake for about 30 minutes, rotating the muffin tin 180° halfway through the cooking process. The muffins are done when a toothpick inserted into the middle comes out clean and the tops feel springy to the touch.

9. Take the muffins out of the oven. Cool the tray on a rack for about 5 minutes and then pop the muffins out and completely cool them directly on the rack.

6. **Easy breakfast casserole**

Ingredients

- 2 tablespoons fat of choice (coconut oil or butter or ghee, etc.), melted
- 1 large sweet potato or yam, diced
- 1/2 teaspoon fine sea salt

- 1 1/2 pound breakfast sausage

- 1/2 yellow onion, diced

- 2 cups chopped spinach

- 10 eggs, whisked

- 1/2 teaspoon salt

- 1/2 teaspoon garlic powder

Instructions

1. Preheat oven to 400 degrees. Grease a 9×12 baking dish.

2. Toss diced sweet potatoes in fat and sprinkle with salt

3. Place sweet potatoes on baking sheet and bake for 20-25 minutes, until soft.

4. While sweet potatoes are cooking, place a large sauté pan over medium heat. Add breakfast sausage and yellow onion. Cook until no pink remains in meat.

5. Place meat mixture in baking dish, add sweet potatoes and spinach then add

eggs along with salt and garlic powder and mix until well combine.

6. Place in oven and bake for 25-30 minutes, until eggs are set in the middle.

7. **Egg bake casserole**

Ingredients

- 2 whole eggs, pastured
- 1/8 cup onion, diced
- 1/8 cup zucchini, halved and sliced
- 1/8 cup broccoli, chopped
- 1/8 cup spinach, chopped
- 1 tsp salt
- 1 tsp coconut oil, organic

Instruction

1. Preheat oven to 350°f.
2. Whisk two eggs in a mixing bowl.

3. Stir in chopped vegetables and sprinkle in salt.

4. Lightly grease a single-serving nonstick soufflé dish with coconut oil.

5. Pour egg mixture into the soufflé dish.

6. Bake at 350°f for 20–25 minutes.

7. Serve.

Notes

A side of fresh fruit, bacon, or sausage will go well with this recipe. You can even get creative and mix cooked sausage or ground meat into the eggs prior to cooking, or top with crumbled bacon.

8. Salmon chowder

Ingredients

Salmon broth

- 3 to 4 pounds salmon heads, fins and bones , gills removed

- salt

- 1 onion, chopped

- 2 carrots, chopped

- 2 celery stalks, chopped

- 1 cup white wine

- 1 handful of dried mushrooms, preferably matsutake

- 2 bay leaves

Chowder

- 1/4 pound thick bacon

- 1 cup chopped yellow or white onion

- 2 celery stalks, chopped

- 1 1/2 pounds potatoes, peeled and diced

- 5 tp 6 cups fish broth, or 4 cups chicken broth plus 1 to 2 cups water

- 1 to 2 pounds skinless, boneless salmon meat, cut into chunks

- 1 cup corn, fresh or thawed

- 2/3 cup heavy cream

- black pepper to taste

- 2 tablespoons chopped fresh dill or chives, for garnish

Instructions

1. To make the broth, put all the broth ingredients into the pot and cover with water. Bring to a bare simmer, or even just let it steep like a tea, for 30 to 45 minutes. Strain the broth. Pick any stray salmon meat you want off the bones and reserve. Discard the rest of the solids and reserve the broth.

2. Wipe out the pot, add the bacon, and turn the heat to medium, and cook the bacon until crispy. Remove the bacon. Eat 1 piece. Chop the rest and reserve.

3. Sauté the onion and celery in the bacon fat, stirring often, until they are soft, about 4 to 5 minutes. Add the potatoes and the salmon broth and bring to a simmer. Add salt to taste. Cook until the potatoes are tender, about 15 to 20 minutes.

4. When the potatoes are tender, add the corn and the chunks of salmon. Cook gently until the salmon is just cooked through, about 5 minutes. Turn off the heat and stir in the chopped bacon, dill, heavy cream and black pepper.

9. Blueberry soup

Ingredients

- 3 cups blueberries, fresh or frozen
- 2 tablespoons honey
- 2 teaspoons lemon juice

- 1 cinnamon stick, optional

- 2 teaspoons cornstarch

- 1 teaspoon lemon zest

- Yogurt for serving, if desired

Instruction

1. Combine the berries with the honey, lemon juice, cinnamon stick if using (it's traditional, but i generally don't use any) and a cup of water.

2. Bring to a gentle boil, then turn down to a low simmer, cover and cook 8-10 minutes, until the berries are stewed. (at this point, it's also traditional to strain the berry skins out and just use the juice, but i like to leave them in for more texture.)

3. Stir the cornstarch into 1 tbs. Of warm water to make a slurry, then stir this into the cooked berries. Bring back to a very gentle boil and cook, stirring, until starting

to thicken, about 2 minutes. Remove from the heat and stir in the lemon zest.

4. Serve warm, or chill and serve later. Top with a scoop of yogurt before serving (or use whipped cream or creme fraiche instead of yogurt if you'd like to make this a dessert).

10. Warming carrot, ginger and turmeric soup

Ingredients

- 3 carrots
- 1 white onion
- 3 cloves garlic minced
- 1 inch piece of fresh ginger finely grated
- 2 inch piece of fresh turmeric finely grated
- 4 cups (950ml) vegetable stock
- 1 tbsp lemon juice
- Canned coconut milk (for topping)

- Black sesame seeds (for topping)

Instructions

1. Dice the onion and carrot into small chunks (no need to be precise as everything will be blended at the end), and grate the ginger and turmeric finely.

2. Heat a small amount of olive oil in the bottom of a large stock pot and saute the onion for 3 minutes until translucent, then add the minced garlic, turmeric and ginger and saute for another 1 minute.

3. Next, add the diced carrot and saute for another 2 minutes. Then add the vegetable stock and simmer for 20-25 minutes until the carrot is cooked through and soft.

4. Use a stick blender to blend the soup until it's smooth, or transfer into a standing blender and blend. Stir in the lemon juice,

then serve with a swirl of coconut milk
and some black sesame seeds.

11. Turkey, kale, and cauliflower soup

Ingredients

- 1 lb. Ground turkey;
- 4 shallots, chopped;
- 3 carrots, sliced;
- 1 bell pepper, cut into pieces;
- 15 oz can diced tomatoes;
- 5 cups chicken stock;
- 1 ½ cup cauliflower, minced;
- 4 cups kale, ribs removed, leaves coarsely chopped;
- 2 tbsp. Coconut oil;
- Sea salt and freshly ground black pepper;

Instruction

1. Melt the coconut oil in a saucepan placed over medium-high heat.

2. Add the shallots, carrots, cauliflower, and bell pepper.

3. Cook until the vegetables are slightly soft (8 to 10 minutes), stirring frequently.

4. Add the turkey to the vegetables and cook until the meat is cooked through (6 to 8 minutes).

5. Add the chicken stock and diced tomatoes, and season with salt and pepper to taste.

6. Bring the soup to a boil. Stir in the kale, reduce the heat to low, and let it simmer, covered, for 15 minutes.

12. Baked super foods: salmon, kale & sweet potatoes

Ingredients

- 1 sweet potato
- 1 bunch kale
- 1 lb. Filet of wild salmon
- 1 orange
- 1 grapefruit
- 1 lemon
- 3 tablespoons olive oil
- 1 ½ tsp. Kosher salt
- 1 ½ tsp. Course ground black pepper
- 1 pat butter
- 12 cherry or grape tomatoes

Instructions

1. I prepared this dish in two single-serve baking dishes. You could also prepare it in one 13 x 9 pan.

2. Julienne the sweet potato into strips. Toss with 1 tablespoon olive oil, 1 tablespoon orange juice, ½ tsp. Orange zest, ½ tsp.

Salt and ½ tsp. Pepper. Place half on one side of each baking dish.

3. Rinse and chop the leafy part of the kale. Toss with 1 tablespoon olive oil, 1 tablespoon grapefruit juice, ½ tsp. Grapefruit zest, ½ tsp. Salt and ½ tsp. Pepper. Place half on the other side of each baking dish.

4. Cut the salmon filet in half. Toss with 1 tablespoon olive oil, 1 tablespoon lemon juice, ½ tsp. Lemon zest, ½ tsp. Salt and ½ tsp. Pepper. Place a filet in each dish between the sweet potatoes and kale, skin side down. Top with a pat of butter and a lemon slice.

5. Place 3 cherry tomatoes on the sides of each filet.

6. Bake in a 400-degree oven for 25 minutes.

13. Chicken piccata

Ingredients

- 2 boneless chicken breasts, butterflied
- 1/3 cup almond flour
- 5 tbsp extra virgin olive oil
- 6 tbsp coconut oil
- 1/3 cup fresh lemon juice
- 1/2 cup low sodium chicken broth
- 1/4 cup capers
- 1/3 cup fresh parsley chopped
- Salt to taste
- Pepper to taste
- 5 oz baby portabella mushrooms sliced

Instructions

1. Season chicken with salt and pepper. Pour almond flour in a bowl and dredge both sides in almond flour, shaking off excess.

2. In a large skillet over medium high heat, melt 2 tablespoons of coconut oil with 3 tablespoons olive oil.

3. When mixture starts to sizzle, add 2 pieces of chicken and cook for 3 minutes (or until browned), flip and cook other side or until browned.

4. Remove and transfer to plate. Melt 2 more tablespoons coconut oil and add another 2 tablespoons olive oil. When this mixture starts to sizzle, add 2 more pieces of chicken and brown both sides as with the first batch.

5. At the same time, add mushrooms and saute for 5 minutes (may need to add a tad more coconut and olive oil). Remove pan from heat, and add chicken to the plate.

6. In the pan, add the lemon juice, stock, and capers. Return to stove and bring to a

boil, scraping up brown bits from pan for extra flavor. Taste to check for seasoning, then return all the chicken to the pan and simmer for 5 minutes. Remove chicken to a serving dish. Add 2 remaining tablespoons of coconut oil to sauce and whisk vigorously. Pour sauce over chicken and garnish with parsley.

7. Serve and enjoy!

14. Baked whitefish with tomatoes & olives

Ingredients

- Two 4-5-ounce whitefish fillets (haddock, cod, pollock whatever you can find at the local fish market), skin and any bones removed

- 2 garlic cloves, crushed

- 1 tbsp extra virgin olive oil

- 1 pint of cherry or grape tomatoes, halved

- 1 tbsp white wine

- 1/4 cup black or kalamata olives, pitted

- Handful of fresh basil, finely chopped

- Slr's spice of life or your favorite seasoning blend

Instruction

1. Preheat oven to 425°

2. Pour the olive oil into a large oven-safe skillet set over medium heat. When shimmering, add the garlic. Cook, stirring often, until garlic is fragrant but not browned, one to two minutes.

3. Add the tomatoes to the skillet. Stir in the white wine. Remove from heat.

4. Season the fish fillets, we prefer to use our own spice of life blend, but you can use whichever salt-free seasoning blend you like best. Place the fish fillets into the

pan so they touch the bottom of the pan. Top the two fillets with the olives and basil leaves. Spoon some of the tomatoes and pan juice over the tops of the fillets.

5. Transfer skillet to the oven and cook until fish is done, 10 to 15 minutes.

6. Serve with sautéed zucchini or summer squash.

15.Slow cooker coconut curry cashew chicken

Ingredients

- 3 boneless skinless chicken breasts - pounded thin and chopped into bite-size pieces
- 1 red pepper - seeded and thinly sliced
- 2 small potatoes - (i used red), peeled and chopped
- ½ white or yellow onion - chopped

- 2 cups chicken broth

- 2 cups unsweetened coconut milk - (or one 14-ounce can + 1/2 cup chicken broth)

- 3 tablespoons yellow curry powder - (see note)

- 1 teaspoon cumin

- 1 teaspoon salt - or to taste

- ½ teaspoon cayenne pepper - or to taste

- Optional: corn starch slurry - (see note)

- Cashews, cilantro, cooked rice for serving

Instructions

1. Add chicken pieces, red peppers, potatoes, and onions to the slow cooker.

2. In a medium bowl whisk together chicken broth, curry powder, cumin, salt, and cayenne pepper. Pour mixture into slow cooker and stir to coat chicken and

veggies. Cover and cook on high for 2-3 hours or on low 4-5 hours.

3. About 10-15 minutes before serving, stir in coconut milk. Stir just before serving and top with cashews and freshly chopped cilantro.

Notes

*if you have red curry paste on hand, i like to swap out 1 tablespoon of curry powder for 1 tablespoon of the red paste. You can also add up to 1 tablespoon of garlic powder for an extra flavor boost. *if you prefer a little bit thicker curry (like i do) whisk together 3 tablespoons cold water and 2 tablespoons corn starch. Stir into crockpot about 30-45 minutes before serving and cook on high until ready to serve.

16. Honey and wasabi glazed salmon

Ingredients

- 4 tbsp apple cider vinegar
- 2 fillet (170g) atlantic salmon, wild
- 1 tbsp coconut aminos, coconut secret
- 1 tbsp coconut oil
- 1 tsp minced ginger root
- 2 tbsp honey
- 2 tsp wasabi powder

Instructions

1. Preheat oven to 425 degrees.
2. In a small sauce pan stir together white wine vinegar, honey, coconut aminos, ginger root and wasabi powder.
3. Bring to a boil and reduce to simmer for 6-8 minutes, or until thickened, stirring occasionally. Set aside.

4. In a large oven-proof skillet, melt your coconut oil on high. Sear the salmon skin side up for about 3 minutes.

5. Turn the fillets, and pour on half the glaze. Place the skillet in the oven for 4-6 minutes, depending on the thickness of the fillet , and your desired done-ness.

6. When cooked, remove the fish from the oven, and pour over the reserved glaze.

17. Beanless chili

Ingredients

- 1 red pepper, diced
- 1 small onion, diced
- 1 small box of sliced mushrooms
- 1 medium zucchini, diced
- 1 pound of grass-fed beef or bison cubes
- 1 teaspoon fresh garlic or equivalent (jar or dried works well, too)

- 1 can tomato paste (6 oz.)
- 1 can tomato sauce (8 oz.)
- 1-1/2 fresh diced tomatoes (or one 14-1/2 oz. Can)
- 1 small can of green chilies (4 oz.)
- 1-1/2 tablespoons chili powder mix
- ½ cup beef broth (homemade is best)
- Pinch of salt
- Pinch of crushed dried red peppers
- 1 teaspoon hot chili sauce
- ½ teaspoon finely chopped jalapeño (optional)

Instructions

1. Place the meat cubes in the pot, then add vegetables and tomato sauce and paste.
2. Mix all seasonings with the beef broth and pour evenly over the top of the vegetables.

3. Cover and cook on low for 7-8 hours or on
   high for 4 hours.

18. Rosemary lemon roasted chicken breasts

Ingredients

- 1-2 medium lemons, sliced

- 2 sprigs rosemary

- 2 cloves garlic , quartered

- 1 pound uncooked boneless skinless chicken breasts

- 1 tablespoon extra virgin olive oil

- 1 teaspoon kosher salt

- 1/2 teaspoon fresh ground black pepper

Instructions

1. Preheat oven to 425°f. Layer 1/2 lemon slices and 1 sprig of rosemary on the

bottom of a baking dish. Scatter 1/2 of
garlic around the pan.

2. Season both sides of chicken with salt and
   pepper. Lay chicken on top of lemon
   rosemary bed.

3. Place remaining lemon slices on top of
   chicken breasts. Place rosemary sprig
   between the chicken breasts. Sprinkle
   with remaining garlic. Drizzle chicken
   breasts with olive oil.

4. Bake for 25-30 minutes until chicken is
   cooked through (1 pound takes about 25-
   30 minutes, 5 pounds takes 45-60
   minutes). Cover with aluminum foil for 5
   minutes and let the chicken rest. Serve
   and enjoy!

Notes

1. You can double, triple, quadruple, etc this
   recipe. I make it with 5 pounds of chicken
   so we have enough to eat all week.

2. If you prefer your chicken more browned
   on top, at the end of your cook time turn
   the broiler on and cook for 2-3 minutes
   until chicken and lemons are browned.

19. Thai curry chicken

Ingredients

1. 1 pound boneless skinless chicken thighs

2. ½ teaspoon diamond crystal brand kosher
   salt

3. Freshly ground black pepper

4. 1 tablespoon coconut oil or fat of choice

5. 1 small onion chopped medium

6. 1-2 tablespoons thai curry paste
   whichever color you prefer

7. 1 cup full-fat coconut milk

8. 10 ounces frozen mixed vegetables

9. 2 cups leftover roasted kabocha squash or
    roasted butternut squash, frozen sweet
    potatoes, etc.

10. 2 tablespoons apple juice optional

11. ¼ cup fresh basil leaves thinly sliced

Instructions

1. Cut the chicken into medium-sized chunks
    and season with salt and pepper.

2. Heat a medium saucepan over medium
    heat until hot. Swirl in the coconut oil.
    When the oil is shimmering, brown the
    chicken and transfer to a separate plate.

3. Add the onions to the saucepan and sauté
    until translucent. Return the chicken and
    juices to the pot, and add the curry paste
    to taste. (start with 1 tablespoon and add
    more if needed later.)

4. Stir-fry until you can smell the rich aroma
    of toasted spices. Pour in the coconut milk
    and toss in the frozen veggies, squash,
    and apple juice (if using).

5. Raise the heat to high and bring the
    contents of the pot to a boil. Then, turn
    the heat down to medium-low and
    simmer the curry for 10 minutes or until
    the veggies are warmed through and the
    flavors meld. Taste for seasoning and
    adjust as needed.

6. Add the basil chiffonade and serve over
    zoodles, plain cauliflower rice, or asian
    cauliflower fried rice.

20. Blackened fish tacos with avocado sauce

Ingredients

- 1 lb. Tilapia fillets or other white-fleshed fish fillets, approximately ¾ - 1 inch thick*
- 2-3 tbsp. Olive oil

Blackened seasoning:

- 1 tsp. Paprika
- ¼ tsp. Garlic powder
- ½ tsp. Black pepper
- 1/8 – ¼ tsp. Cayenne pepper depending on your spice preference
- ¼ tsp. Oregano dried
- ¾ tsp. Salt

Avocado sauce:

- 1 large avocado peeled and pitted
- 2 tbsp. Greek yogurt or dairy-free, plain
- 2 tbsp. Lime juice fresh
- 2 tbsp. Cilantro plus more for serving
- ¼ tsp. Salt

Serving:

- 8 corn tortillas*

- ½ cup cabbage shredded

- ¼ cup cilantro finely chopped

- ¼ cup green onions chopped

- ¼ cup queso fresco crumbled, optional

- See this recipe in meal plan #5

Instructions

1. In a small bowl combine blackened seasoning ingredients. Toss to combine.

2. Sprinkle blackened seasoning over both sides of the fish fillets. Rub seasoning into the fillets.

3. Place 2-3 tablespoons of oil into a cast iron skillet over medium-low heat. Add fish fillets to heated skillet and cook for 4-5 minutes on both sides.*

4. While fish fillets are cooking, place avocado, yogurt, lime juice, 2 tablespoons cilantro, and ¼ teaspoon of salt into a

small food processor or blender. Process until completely smooth and thoroughly combined.

5. Serve cooked fish on corn tortillas* with avocado sauce, cabbage, additional cilantro, green onions and queso fresca.

Notes

If you choose another type of fish with a thickness greater than ¾ - 1 inch, be sure to cook the fish for additional time to ensure they are completely cooked.

Warm up your corn tortillas in a skillet with a bit of coconut oil for added flavor.

21. Salmon and beet salad with spicy dressing

Ingredients

- 6 oz. Cooked or canned salmon, flaked;

- 3 cups lettuce;

- ¼ avocado, diced;

- ½ grapefruit or 1 large orange, roughly chopped;

- ¼ small red onion, thinly sliced;

- ½ cup cooked beets, diced;

- 10 pistachio nuts, shelled and chopped;

22. Salmon and beet salad recipe

Ingredients

- 6 oz. Cooked or canned salmon, flaked;

- 3 cups lettuce;

- ¼ avocado, diced;

- ½ grapefruit or 1 large orange, roughly chopped;

- ¼ small red onion, thinly sliced;

- ½ cup cooked beets, diced;

- 10 pistachio nuts, shelled and chopped;

Ingredients for spicy dressing

- 1 tbsp. Extra-virgin olive oil;
- 2 tbsp. Fresh orange juice;
- 2 tsp. White wine vinegar;
- ½ tsp. Orange zest;
- ½ tsp. Dijon or homemade mustard;
- ½ or ¼ tsp. Chili powder;
- Sea salt and freshly ground black pepper to taste;

Instruction

1. In a small bowl, combine all the ingredients for the dressing and whisk until smooth. Season to taste.
2. In a large bowl, combine the salmon, lettuce, avocado, grapefruit or orange, onion, and beets.
3. Drizzle the dressing on top of the salad and toss well.

4. Sprinkle the pistachio on top of the salad and serve.

23.Supercharged coconut curry

ingredients

- 1 can full fat coconut milk
- 1 ½ cup of organic chicken broth
- 2 cups of stir-fry veggies: broccoli, carrots and cauliflower
- 1 cup of diced up bell peppers
- 1 cup of diced up red onions
- ½ tsp of pink salt & taste of black pepper
- 2 ½ tbsp. Of red curry paste
- 4-5 cloves of minced garlic
- Juice of one lime
- 3 tbsps. Of grass-fed butter, ghee or coconut oil
- 1 tsp of turmeric
- 1 cup of kale or spinach

- 2 cups of shredded organic chicken or grass-fed beef

- 1 head of cauliflower to make cauliflower rice

Instructions

1. start by cooking the meat of your choice.

2. remove the cooked meat and set a side in a bowl.

3. add the coconut milk and chicken stock to a large pot along with the curry paste, butter, turmeric, lime, garlic. Cook for 5 minutes, stirring occasionally.

4. then add the frozen or fresh veggie mixes to the pot, stir, and cover while cooking for 5 minutes. If you added sweet potato, cook until soft.

5. remove the lid and stir in the chicken, beef, or beans. Cover and cook for the last 5 minutes.

6. serve over a bowl of cauliflower rice or by itself.

7. place head of cauliflower in blender and pulse until it turns into the consistency of rice.

8. either saute on low heat in coconut oil until soft, or steam until it becomes the softness you wish (does not take long).

24. Crock pot mocha pot roast

Ingredients

- 2 tbsp finely ground coffee beans
- 2 tbsp smoked paprika
- 1 tbsp black pepper
- 1 tbsp cocoa powder
- 1 tsp aleppo pepper or sweet paprika
- 1 tsp chili powder
- 1 tsp ground ginger
- 1 tsp sea salt

- For the roast

- 2 lb beef roast i used grass-fed chuck

- 1 cup brewed coffee

- 1 cup beef broth

- 1/2 an onion chopped

- 6 dried figs chopped

- 3 tbsp balsamic vinegar

Instructions

1. Prepare the mocha rub by mixing together the finely ground coffee, smoked paprika, black pepper, cocoa powder, aleppo pepper (sub: sweet paprika), chili powder, ground ginger and salt in a small bowl. You won't use the entire batch if you're making a 2-pound roast. It stores well in an airtight container.

2. Pat the beef roast dry with a paper towel. Spoon 3 to 4 tablespoons of the mocha

rub mixture over the roast and rub it in well with your hands.

3. Combine the brewed coffee, beef broth, onion, figs, and balsamic vinegar in a blender. Puree until liquified.

4. Pour the liquid into the crock pot and place the roast gently on top.

5. Cook for 5 to 6 hours on low.

6. Remove the meat and shred with two forks. You can then boil the liquid until it reduces and thickens or simply serve as is. Adjust seasonings with salt and pepper to taste.

25. Creamy dill and garlic salmon

Ingredients

- 2 salmon fillets pinbones removed

- 1/2 cup homemade mayonnaise

- 2 tablespoons fresh dill chopped

- 2 teaspoons brown mustard

- 1 clove garlic finely minced

- Pinch of sea salt

Instructions

1. Preheat oven to 450 degrees and line a baking sheet with parchment paper.
2. Place salmon fillets, skin side down, on the paper.
3. Mix mayonnaise, dill, mustard, garlic, and salt.
4. Spread mixture evenly over salmon and bake for 8-10 minutes, or just until flesh flakes under your fork.
5. Serve hot with a squeeze of fresh lemon.

26. Coconut curry salmon

Ingredients

Salmon:

- 1 1/2 lbs. Salmon

- 1 tablespoon brown sugar

- 1 teaspoon curry powder

- 1/2 teaspoon onion powder

- 1/2 teaspoon garlic powder

- 1/2 teaspoon kosher salt (more for a larger filet)

- 1–2 teaspoons olive oil

Coconut curry sauce:

- 1 tablespoon olive oil

- 2 cloves garlic (minced)

- 1 small knob of ginger (minced)

- 1 tablespoon of lemongrass paste

- 1 tablespoon brown sugar

- 1 tablespoon red curry paste

- 1 can coconut milk

- 2 tablespoons fish sauce or soy sauce

- Lots of lime juice and zest

- 3 cups fresh spinach, chopped

For serving:

- Cilantro, basil, mint, or other fresh herbs
- Rice
- Cook mode prevent your screen from going dark

Instructions

1. Get the oven ready: preheat the oven to 475 degrees. Line a baking sheet with foil. Place one of the oven racks close-ish to the top, about 6 inches or so.
2. Make your rice: cook rice according to package instructions.
3. Salmon: mix the spices and the olive oil to make a paste. Place the salmon skin side down on the baking sheet. Rub the paste liberally over the top part of the salmon. Bake for 6-12 minutes (depends on salmon thickness and desired doneness – i usually opt for 8-10 minutes). See notes

and faqs for potential broiling issues and alternative methods.

4. Coconut curry sauce: heat the olive oil over medium heat. Add garlic, ginger, and lemongrass; sauté for 5 minutes.

5. Add brown sugar and curry paste; sauté for 3 minutes. Add coconut milk. Season with fish sauce and lime juice to taste. Add spinach; stir into the sauce until wilted.

6. Serve: place salmon over rice. Cover with sauce, lime juice, and fresh herbs.

Notes

If you try broiling the salmon, it can work (i have done it many times) but it is possible for your salmon, when rubbed with the sugar mixture, to light on fire if you get it too close to the heating element of your oven. If you are concerned about this, i would just use the regular oven temp of 450/475 as directed and wait until the oven has preheated to put your salmon in.